Melanie Tamara Carolin Kuffner

Mechanisms of Adaptation and Reconstruction in the Hypoperfused Brain

Melanie Tamara Carolin Kuffner

MECHANISMS OF ADAPTATION AND RECONSTRUCTION IN THE HYPOPERFUSED BRAIN

Bibliografische Information der Deutschen Nationalbibliothek: Die Deutsche Nationalbibliothek verzeichnet diese Publikation in der Deutschen Nationalbibliografie; detaillierte bibliografische Daten sind im Internet über http://dnb.dnb.de abrufbar.

Die automatisierte Analyse des Werkes, um daraus Informationen insbesondere über Muster, Trends und Korrelationen gemäß §44b UrhG („Text und Data Mining") zu gewinnen, ist untersagt.

© 2024 Melanie Tamara Carolin Kuffner

Verlag: BoD · Books on Demand GmbH, In de Tarpen 42, 22848 Norderstedt

Druck: Libri Plureos GmbH, Friedensallee 273, 22763 Hamburg

ISBN: 978-3-7597-4874-4

Melanie Tamara Carolin Kuffner
Mechanisms of Adaptation and Reconstruction in the Hypoperfused Brain

Table of Contents

List of abbreviations 3
Abstract 5
1. Introduction 7
  1.1 Current state of research 7
    1.1.1 Burden of disease 7
    1.1.2 Pathophysiology in ischemic settings 8
    1.1.3 IL-6 in the ischemic brain 10
    1.1.4 SorCS2 and astrocytes 11
  1.2 Objective 13
2. Methods 15
  2.1 Animals and mouse models 15
  2.2 In vivo design 18
  2.3 Western blotting and ELISA 20
  2.4 Cell culture and transfection 21
  2.5 RT-qPCR 22
  2.6 Laser capture microdissection 23
  2.7 Immunohistochemistry 23
  2.8 Image analysis 25
  2.9 Statistical analyses 26
  2.10 Methods to prevent bias 26

3. **Results** 27

    3.1   IL-6 mediates brain remodeling after unilateral CCAo 27

    3.2   SorCS2 is secreted by astrocytes and regulates endostatin after stroke 31

    3.3   A data driven approach using machine learning provides humane endpoints in murine stroke models 34

4. **Discussion** 39

    4.1   Summary, interpretation and embedding into the state of the art research 40

    4.2   Strengths and weaknesses 45

5. **Conclusions** 49

Reference List 51

List of abbreviations

ANOVA	analysis of variance
BBB	blood-brain barrier
CCAo	occlusion of common carotid artery
DALY	Disability-adjusted life year
DAPI	4',6-diamidino-2-phenylindole
EGFP	enhanced green fluorescent protein
ELISA	enzyme-linked immunosorbent assay
FLEX	flip-excision
GABA	γ-aminobutyric acid
GFAP	glial fibrillary acidic protein
GAPDH	glyceraldehyde 3-phosphate dehydrogenase
IGFBP3	insulin-like growth factor-binding protein 3
IFNγ	interferon gamma
IL	interleukin
LCM	laser capture microdissection
LTP	long-term potentiation
MAPK/ERK	mitogen-activated protein kinase
MCAo	occlusion of the middle cerebral artery
mRNA	messenger ribonucleic acid

PFA	paraformaldehyde
PMA	phorbol 12-myristate 13-acetate
PBS	phosphate-buffered saline
RT-qPCR	reverse transcription polymerase chain reaction
SorCS2	sortilin-related Vps10p domain containing receptor 2
SIRS	systemic inflammatory response syndrome
TGF-β1	transforming growth factor beta 1
VECdh	vascular endothelial cadherin
VEGF	vascular endothelial growth factor

Melanie Tamara Carolin Kuffner
Mechanisms of Adaptation and Reconstruction in the Hypoperfused Brain

Abstract

Ischemic damage to the brain poses a long-term disability or even death. Endogenous recovery cannot fully restore functionality by itself, leading to deficits in cognition and motor function. This thesis investigates microenvironmental changes mediated by the molecules interleukin 6 (IL-6) and SorCS2 in murine models of ischemia.

Our first study focuses on the effect of the inflammatory cytokine IL-6 in carotid stenosis, evaluating changes in the brain parenchyma and other associated factors. IL-6 plays an ambivalent role in the hypoperfused brain: it is associated with poor outcome such as deterioration in motor function, but it is also essential for recovery processes. In this study, mice underwent unilateral carotid artery occlusion, and IL-6 overexpression in astrocytes was induced on day 2 after surgery. Motor skills and health status were monitored for 21 days using behavioral tests, and changes in cerebral connectivity and brain remodeling were examined using diffusion tensor imaging. Data analysis showed that IL-6 overexpression has no adverse effect on the overall condition and fosters connectivity changes in the brain. In total, 10 out of 14 tracts were increased, mainly in interhemispheric networks. Proteome analysis of the ipsilesional striatal fiber tracts and the contralesional motor cortex showed alterations in expression levels of plasticity-associated proteins. Caprin-1 was more abundantly expressed on the ipsilesional side, and the GABA-transporter Gat1 was downregulated on the contralesional side, reducing inhibitory GABA signaling. Both are targets for further studies and potential drug targets for translatory research.

The second part of the thesis investigates the effects of a SorCS2 knockout in stroke models. This Vps10p sorting receptor is a regulator of vesicular trafficking and secretion, possibly involved in endogenous IL-6 regulation. The study showed that contrary to prior knowledge, not only neurons but also astrocytes express SorCS2 after stroke, and TGF-β likely mediates induction. IL-6 was not confirmed to be regulated in *in vivo* assays. Ablation of SorCS2 correlated with endostatin expression, mediating effects on regenerative processes such as angiogenesis.

Our third study focuses on improving animal research. Data from standardized behavioral tests were collected in one curated database. This allows meta-analysis of data and can reduce animal suffering and the number of experimental animals due to higher experimental standards and prediction of human endpoints. It also generated a new starting point for innovative research concepts based on existing animal data.

In summary, the thesis contributes insights into post-ischemic recovery processes and found several potential targets for further research on therapeutic interventions for brain ischemia. It also contributes to the 3R approach of reducing animal suffering in experimental research.

1. Introduction

1.1 Current state of research

1.1.1 Burden of disease

The industrialized world is characterized by increasingly aging societies and the rise of age-related diseases, most prominently dementia, heart attacks, and stroke. Cardiovascular diseases attribute to over a third of all deaths in Germany, and cerebrovascular diseases alone are the fifth leading cause of death in the United States.[1,2] Considering the combined cause of death and disability, stroke ranks third globally.[3] Carotid artery occlusion is highly linked to stroke and is attributable to patients' cognitive impairment.[4,5] The burden of disease is tremendous, and additionally to implementing preventive measures, new therapy options and medication are needed to improve patients' lives and unburden health care systems.

In stroke, therapy focuses on revascularization – only applicable for a small subset of patients – and physical rehabilitation therapy.[6] Major impairments, especially of general motor function, still affect stroke patients massively in their everyday lives with a high count of disability-adjusted life years (DALYs).[7,8] Carotid stenosis treatment usually consists of carotid endarterectomy, stenting, or medical therapy focusing on halting disease progression and preventing stroke. Despite the high prevalence of ischemic events, there are no or very few efficient pharmacological treatment options that concentrate on the recovery from ischemic stroke and the consequences of chronic hypoperfusion due to stenosis. This is attributable to the only partly understood and very complex interplay of processes in the ischemic brain.

1.1.2 Pathophysiology in ischemic settings

Stroke and carotid artery occlusion both lead to pathophysiological mechanisms and brain damage, such as white matter lesions and, in stroke, brain atrophy. Long-term or severe short-term hypoperfusion of the brain leads to a lack of oxygen and glucose, especially in the watershed regions of the brain. In stroke, this leads to a profound change in the cerebral microenvironment by activating the so-called ischemic cascade, a complex process involving excitotoxicity, oxidative stress, blood-brain barrier (BBB) dysfunction, activation of the immune system, and cell death.[9] In carotid artery occlusion and accompanying chronic cerebral hypoperfusion, the stress on the brain cells is less pronounced, leading to slower pathophysiology. The main hallmarks found in hypoperfusion models are white matter damage, blood-brain barrier disruption, and mild astrogliosis, ultimately speculated to lead to vascular dementia.[10–13]

Ameliorating brain recovery is an attractive target for the treatment of ischemic diseases. The brain can re-establish parts of functionality lost due to insufficient perfusion. Intact areas of the brain can compensate missing function. This is called plasticity. New neuronal connections form between previously unconnected regions and enable the re-establishment of function.[14] The underlying mechanisms are only partially known. Among the contributors fostering plasticity, besides neurogenesis, are angiogenesis, extracellular matrix remodeling, and inflammatory cues.[15–18] There has been a strong focus on investigating brain composition changes after and during ischemia to better understand beneficial and detrimental processes. The critical processes for recovery, angiogenesis and inflammation, are both ambivalent and can influence one another via signaling molecules such as vascular endothelial growth factor (VEGF) for angiogenesis and cytokines such as interleukin (IL)-1β and IL-6.[15,19–22]

1.1.3 IL-6 in the ischemic brain

Inflammation after stroke and ischemia is a complex process initiated by several inflammatory cues and can lead to beneficial and detrimental effects. The glial response to inflammatory cytokines – especially astrogliosis – is necessary in stroke response but can worsen the cognitive function when present excessively.[23,24] Astrogliosis is initiated by circulating cytokines, mainly of the IL-6 family. They activate astrocytes that, in response, express the marker glial fibrillary acidic protein (GFAP) and form the glial scar demarcating the lesioned area.[25–27]

Considering the crucial role of inflammation in ischemic diseases, this thesis primarily focuses on the inflammatory cytokine IL-6. In a non-ischemic setting, IL-6 levels in the bloodstream correlate to sickness severity in mice and humans.[28,29] Constitutive expression of astrocytic IL-6 in non-ischemic mice causes microglial activation and motor deficits.[30] Systemic overexpression of IL-6 in the entire bloodstream is possible with the mouse model presented in this thesis when crossbred with animals carrying the recombinase Cre-ERT2 under control of the endothelial promoter VECdh (Vascular endothelial cadherin). After induction of systemic IL-6, mice rapidly developed symptoms that resemble a cytokine storm and systemic inflammatory response syndrome (SIRS) in humans. These mice showed sickness behavior, leukocytosis, reduced body temperature, splenomegaly, and died.

Local and chronically increased cerebral IL-6 lead to motor deficits in non-ischemic mice.[31] Conversely, IL-6 in the brain has been associated with neuroplasticity.[32,33] In stroke patients, high systemic and cerebrospinal fluid IL-6 levels correlate with poor outcome and higher sickness scores.[34,35] Similarly, in carotid artery stenosis, high serum IL-6 are linked to unfavorable outcome and a higher likelihood of plaque rupture.[36,37] Complete removal of IL-6 in the ischemic mouse brain led to a decrease in angiogenesis, and an overall worsened outcome.[38] These conflicting data hint at an ambivalent role of IL-6 in the ischemic brain. Recovery and plasticity mechanisms possibly depend on exclusively local, paracrine-acting, and moderate levels of IL-6 in the brain, while systemic, high levels might be detrimental to recovery.

1.1.4 SorCS2 and astrocytes

In addition to understanding the effects of IL-6 in ischemic recovery, this thesis addresses the endogenous regulation of signaling molecules after stroke by a specific sorting receptor. Sortilin-related

Vps10p domain containing receptor 2 (SorCS2) is a protein found primarily in neurons in the brain and is part of the Vps10p domain receptors gene family.[39] These receptors play a role in neurotrophin sorting and shuttling, integral for mediating neuronal survival.[40,41] SorCS2 is relevant in psychiatric diseases and was shown to be critical in memory formation and synaptic plasticity.[42,43] Its protective role in oxidative stress models for epilepsy also made it an exciting target for studies in ischemic stroke settings. Similar effects might be observed that favor beneficial outcome.[44] There is limited research on which proteins are interacting and regulated by SorCS2 and are therefore responsible for these beneficial effects. IL-6 is a potential target protein regulated by SorCS2, as others have shown that another member of Vps10p receptors, SorLA, binds IL-6 and mediates its cellular uptake.[45]

1.2 Objective

The primary goals of this study were to investigate beneficial and detrimental factors in the recovery process of stroke and carotid artery occlusion and shed light on crucial recovery mechanisms and active molecules in an exploratory approach. Special attention was given to the use of standardized behavioral protocols and the conceptualization of a unified database for animal data to foster reproducibility of research and open the possibility to re-use data for advanced animal meta-studies.

To this end, the following approaches were taken.

Firstly, the study focused on IL-6 mediated effects on the brain parenchyma in the short-term outcome after carotid artery occlusion. A new mouse model with inducible brain exclusive IL-6 secretion was established and validated. Behavioral, molecular, and connectivity alterations were studied to understand molecular mechanisms and investigate potential new treatment targets for carotid artery occlusion.

Secondly, the role of SorCS2, a sorting receptor, in stroke recovery was studied. We examined expression patterns and means of induction, and functional implications of endogenous SorCS2 upregulation.

Lastly, data-gathering and storage were unified for behavioral studies in ischemic mouse models. Tests, time points, and parameter collection were standardized, and existing data were processed into one single database to allow the re-use of animal data. On this data set, algorithms were trained using machine learning to predict humane endpoints in behavioral mouse stroke studies. This contributes to the efforts of Charité's 3R to improve animal research.

2. Methods

All methods used in this study are described in the publications in detail. This section gives a summary of study designs and critical methods. Details on materials and methods can be found in the respective section of the individual publications (Publication 1: Kuffner et al.[46], Publication 2: Malik et al.[44], Publication 3: Mei et al. [47]).

2.1 Animals and mouse models

Local authorities (Landesamt für Gesundheit und Soziales, (LaGeSo), Berlin (Reg G0119/16, G0157/17)) approved all experimental animal procedures that were conducted in line with German animal protection law and animal welfare guidelines. Mice were kept in groups on a 12 h light/dark cycle and allowed *ad libitum* access to water and food. Animals in behavioral studies had limited food access for 3 h per day with an additional 1.1 g chow overnight to prevent excessive weight loss.

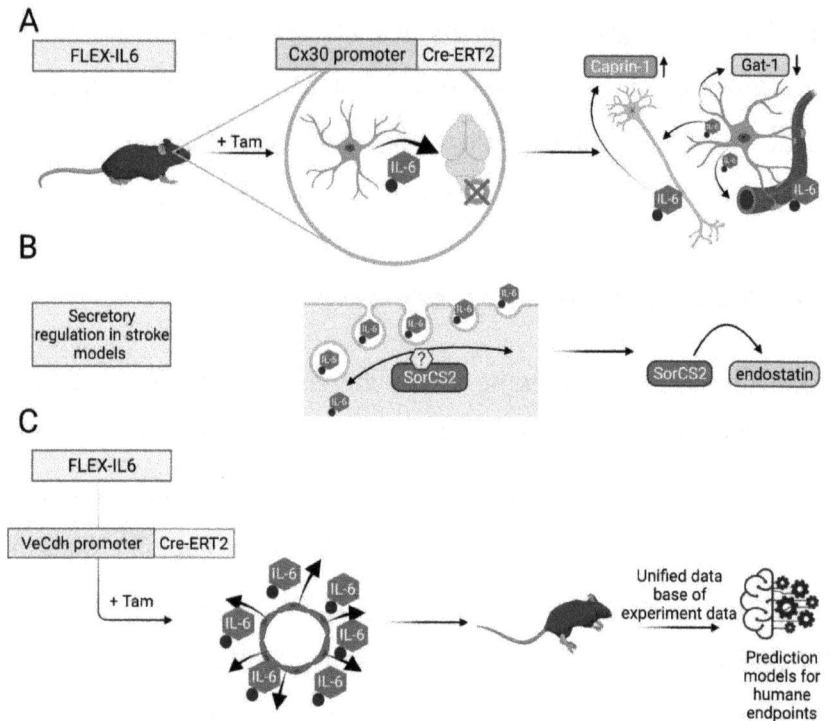

Figure 1 Visual summary of the thesis.

A. Cx30-Cre-ERT2 FLEX-IL6 mouse model with inducible IL-6 expression by tamoxifen administration was used to study the effects of IL-6 in unilateral carotid artery occlusion. Caprin-1 upregulation and Gat1 downregulation were observed in the microenvironmental proteome analysis and can be potential targets for further studies. Additionally, MRI studies showed enhanced connectivity in IL-6 overexpressing animals.

B. The effects of SorCS2 ablation in astrocytes are a potential endogenous regulation mechanism of IL-6. The study showed that mainly endostatin is regulated and at least partially responsible for the recovery effects of SorCS2 after stroke.

C. Mice of the VeCdh-Cre-ERT2 FLEX-IL6 line inducibly express IL-6 in all endothelial cells. The resulting high IL-6 levels lead to severe deterioration and death. The study endpoint for sick mice was challenging to determine, as classical endpoints were not well suited for this scenario. We aimed to find humane endpoints by a data-driven approach to prevent unnecessary animal suffering. We gathered animal data into one large database to re-use data and reduce the number of animals. A novel machine learning based meta-analysis algorithm trained on that data can predict humane endpoints for early termination of the behavioral experiment and reduces animal suffering.

A custom strain of mice was generated for the experiments in publication 1, Cx30-Cre-ERT2; FLEX-IL6 (*Figure 1*). A DNA sequence consisting of murine IL-6, linked by a spacer to a myc-tag, followed by a T2A self-cleavage site, and the fluorescent protein mKate2 was designed. This sequence was embedded in a flip-excision (FLEX) cassette integrated into the R26 locus of mice. The FLEX-IL6 mice were then crossbred with mice carrying an astrocyte-specific Cre-ERT2 recombinase (Cx30-Cre-ERT2). All mice were bred on a C57BL/6J background and used after backcrossing for more than 10 generations. Hemizygous Cx30-Cre-ERT2; FLEX-IL6 mice, or FLEX-IL6 mice at the age of 10 – 12 weeks at the time of surgery were used for the experiments.

In study 2, the mouse line with SorCS2 deletion has been previously described by Glerup et al.[42] and male animals at the age of 8 – 14 weeks at the time of temporary occlusion of the middle cerebral artery (MCAo) have been used for the experiments.

2.2 In vivo design

In publication 1, mice were set on a food-restricted diet with limited food access for 3 h per day four weeks before surgery. Three weeks before surgery, mice started pre-training for the staircase skilled pellet reaching test. Unilateral occlusion of common carotid artery (CCA) was performed by permanently ligating the left CCA (CCAo). One day after surgery, mice were scanned using T2-weighted MRI for visible signs of a stroke or immediate lesions and, in this case, excluded following the preset exclusion criteria. On day two after surgery, animals received i.p. injections of 1 mg tamoxifen (Sigma, 10 mg/ml in 1:10 ethanol/corn oil (all purchased from Sigma)) for one to three consecutive days. Behavioral testing continued two days after surgery. Sickness was evaluated using a modified deSimoni's Neuroscore on days 2, 7, 14, and 21 after surgery. Rotarod testing was done on days 2, 7, and 14 after CCAo in three runs per trial. Staircase pellet reaching was continued daily until 21 days after surgery. On day 21, diffusion tensor imaging (DTI) and T2-weighted MRI were performed. All mice were perfused transcardially on day 21.

In publication 2, animals were subjected to a 45-minute MCAo) as described and observed for short-term (1 and 3 days) or long-term (21 days) studies.[48]

2.3 Western blotting and ELISA

In study 1, serum IL-6 was analyzed using enzyme-linked immunosorbent assay (ELISA) (Mouse IL-6 Quantikine, R&D Systems). Samples were taken from blood sampled on day 5 after surgery and day 3 after induction with tamoxifen.

Brain IL-6 was determined semi-quantitatively by western blotting of homogenized brain tissue. Briefly, deep-frozen brain tissue was homogenized in a rotor-stator homogenizer, centrifuged, and the supernatant treated with detergents to break the cell structure. Samples were treated with ultrasound, and protein content was quantified using Pierce Reagent (Thermo Fisher). The samples were then denatured in reducing sample buffer and separated on 4-12 % SDS-polyacrylamide gels (15-wells, Life Technologies) and subsequently blotted onto a nitrocellulose membrane. After formaldehyde-fixation and washing, proteins were detected using the ReadyTector® system (CANDOR Bioscience; Anti-Mouse-HRP and Anti-Rabbit-HRP) and anti-IL-6 (1:1000, ab6672, Abcam) and anti-GAPDH (1:1000, MAB374, Merck/Millipore) antibodies. Bands were imaged using WesternBright ECL HRP substrate (Advansta) and imager (Vilber Lourmat).

In study 2, brain homogenates were analyzed using the following assays: TGF-β1 (Abcam, ab119557), GFAP (Millipore, NS830), endostatin (Boster, EK1376), U-Plex Biomarker Group 1 assay (Meso Scale Diagnostics, K15083K).

For western blotting, tissue and cell homogenates were studied using the following antibodies: anti-SorCS2 (R&D Systems, AF4237, 1:1,000), anti-p-ERK (Cell Signaling, 4370, 1:2,000), anti-actin (Abcam, ab8227, 1:2,000), anti-GFAP (Millipore, MAB360, 1:1,000). Imaging was performed with the digital LI-COR imaging system.

2.4 Cell culture and transfection

HEK293T cells (Biocat GmbH) were cultured in Dulbecco's Modified Eagle's Medium (DMEM; Gibco) supplemented with 10 % fetal calf serum, 1 % penicillin/streptomycin (Merck), 1 % sodium pyruvate (Gibco), 1 % MEM non-essential amino acids (Gibco) and 1 % GlutaMAX (Gibco). Brain microvascular endothelial cells (bEnd.3, ATCC CRL-2299) were cultured in DMEM (ATCC) supplemented with 1 % L-glutamine (Gibco) and 1 % penicillin/streptomycin (Merck).

For IL-6 production, HEK cells were transfected with plasmids that encode the FLEX-IL6 construct and Cre-EGFP or exclusively the Cre-EGFP plasmid as control using XtremeGene (Roche). After 24 h, the supernatant was harvested and spun down to clear away cellular debris. Murine bEnd.3 cells were incubated with this supernatant from HEK cells transfected with both plasmids or only the control plasmid for 1 h.

2.5 RT-qPCR

Quantitative reverse transcription polymerase chain reaction (RT-qPCR) was performed on bEnd.3 cells after mRNA extraction using random primers and oligo-dT primers (Eurofins) for reverse transcription. Quantitative PCR reaction was done with exon-spanning primers for tyrosine 3-monooxygenase/tryptophan 5-monooxygenase activation protein (Ywhaz) and intron-spanning primers for Il6 using SYBR Green (Qiagen) (Il6 primer sequences: forward GGAAATTGGGGTAGGAAGGAC, reverse ACTTCACAAGTCGGAGGCTT) in study 1 and human samples in study 2. Alterations in mRNA expression levels were calculated using the ddCT method. SorCS2 transcript levels are calculated relative to EF1α. In study 2, murine samples were analyzed with Taqman Gene Expression Assays: Actb (actin, Mm02619580), Col18a1 (collagen XVIII, Mm00487131), GAPDH (Mm99999915), and SorCS2 (Mm00473050). Col18a1 and SorCS2 transcript levels are relative to beta-actin or glyceraldehyde 3-phosphate dehydrogenase (GAPDH).

2.6 Laser capture microdissection

Fiber tracts of the left hemisphere ipsilateral to the occluded artery were isolated using laser capture microdissection (LCM) five days after CCAo and three days after a single tamoxifen dose from fresh frozen tissue fixed in -20 °C acetone/methanol (1:1). Samples were dissolved in 5 M guanidinium-HCl (Serva) and their proteome was analyzed.

2.7 Immunohistochemistry

For histological, biochemical, and proteome analysis, mice were sacrificed by transcardial perfusion in deep anesthesia (100 µl Ketamine/Xylazine (0.7 % Ketamine (10 %, cb pharma), 0.8 % Xylazine (20 mg/ml Xylavet, cb pharma)) per 10 g body weight, i.p.). Blood was sampled from the vena cava, analyzed (scil Vet abc animal blood counter, scil animal care company, Viernheim, Germany; mouse program), left to clot for 30 min, and spun down for 30 min at 4 °C at 290 xg to generate serum. Mice were perfused using 0.9 % saline water.

For proteome analysis, protease inhibitor was added to the perfusion medium (cOmplete™, Roche). Subsequently, mouse brains were taken out, deep-frozen in -45 °C cold 2-methyl butane, and stored at -80 °C until further processing.

For LCM and immunohistochemistry, tissue was cut into 20 µm thick slices with a cryostat (Leica) and fixed in -20 °C acetone/methanol (1:1). Sections were stained overnight and counterstained using 4',6-diamidino-2-phenylindole (DAPI). To reduce background fluorescence, sudan black treatment was applied before mounting. Imaging was carried out on a Leica SP8 confocal microscope using LAS X software on a 20x objective (HC PL APO CS2).

In study 2, mice were perfused transcardially with a solution of DyLight488-labeled lectin (#DL-1174 Vectorlab; 1 mg/ml; 4 µl/g bodyweight) for 180 s followed by 4 % paraformaldehyde (PFA) in phosphate-buffered saline (PBS). This was followed by 24 h post-fixation in 4 % PFA and 36 h in 30 % sucrose/PBS for cryoprotection and snap-frozen in isopentane before sectioning.

The following primary antibodies were used for staining:

Anti-Caprin-1(ab244360, Abcam, 1:200), anti-GAT-1(NBP1-59878, Novus Biologicals, 1:200), anti-GFAP (C9205, Sigma, 1:1,000, coupled to Cy3, for mouse tissue and cells), anti-GFAP (monoclonal mouse, Sigma, 1:4,000, for human tissue), anti-Myc-Tag (9B11)(2233, Cell Signaling, 1:100, coupled to Alexa647), anti-NeuN (MAB377B, Merck/Millipore, 1:100 and 1:200, for murine tissue), anti-NeuN (MAB377 (clone A60), Millipore, 1:2,000, for human tissue), anti-SorCS2 (R&D Systems, AF4237, 1:100, for mouse tissue and cells; anti-SorCS2, Lifespan Biosciences, LS-C501334, 1:450, for human tissue).

2.8 Image analysis

In study 2, the lesion size of stroked animals was determined in images of NeuN, GFAP, and DAPI stained tissue sections using ImageJ software. The respective area was selected manually and measured. The blood vessel area was analyzed using Cell Profiler software. The length of blood vessels was determined manually using the NeuronJ plugin of ImageJ.

2.9 Statistical analyses

GraphPad Prism version 8.2.0 was used for statistical analysis and graphs. Data are shown as scatter dot plots with the mean ± standard deviation with P-values of <0.05 set as significant. Details for the tests used can be found in the respective publication's figure legends. Where normality could be assumed, t-tests, one- and two-way analyses of variance (ANOVA) with Sidak's posthoc comparisons were applied. Outlier analysis was performed using Grubb's and ROUT tests, and outliers were excluded subsequently.

2.10 Methods to prevent bias

All experimenters were blinded to the genotype during the experiments and analysis to prevent bias. Surgery was performed in a random order within a group of mice.

3. Results

3.1 IL-6 mediates brain remodeling after unilateral CCAo

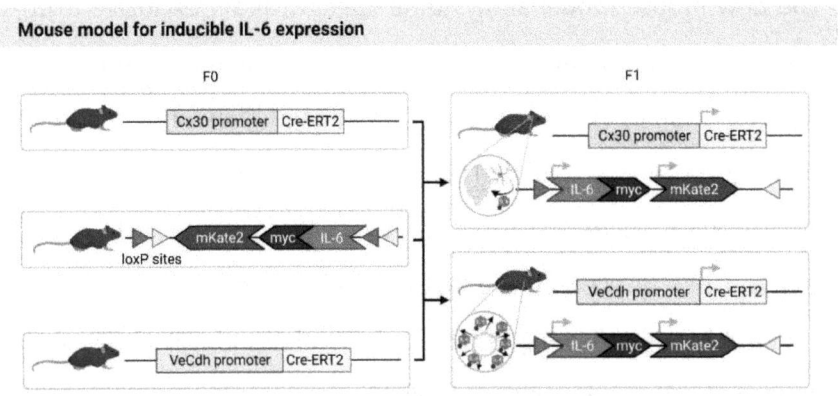

Figure 2 Mouse models used in study 1. The mouse model for inducible secretion of IL-6 uses an inverted FLEX cassette flanked by two different loxP sites inserted into the R26 locus. The FLEX cassette encodes IL-6 linked to a myc-tag and after a self-cleavage site mKate2. Upon recombination by Cre recombinase, the cassette is inverted irreversibly due to the excision of the second loxP site. This model uses the tamoxifen-inducible recombinase Cre-ERT2 for induction at any chosen time point. To achieve tissue specificity, FLEX-Il6 mice are cross-bred with mice that express Cre-ERT2 under the control of either the promotor Cx30 for brain-specific IL-6 secretion by astrocytes or VeCdh for systemic IL-6 secretion in all endothelial cells.

In the first study, the main results comprise the analysis of brain-exclusive IL-6 increase and the effects on CCAo recovery using a newly generated mouse model.[46]

The new mouse model allows time-specific, brain-exclusive expression of IL-6 as a paracrine-acting cytokine. It had an inverted FLEX-cassette coding for IL-6 linked to a myc-tag followed by a T2A self-cleavage sequence and the fluorescent protein mKate2 (*Figure 2; Publication 1, Figure 1A*). Crossbreeding with Cx30-Cre-ERT2 mice resulted in the desired mouse line in which there is a brain-exclusive increase in IL-6 following tamoxifen administration. This was shown by assessing IL-6 expression in brain homogenate by western-blotting and in blood by ELISA (*Publication 1, Figure 1B-D*), with IL-6 increasing significantly in the brain after a single dose compared to controls, but not in serum samples. This mouse line was then used to analyze the effects of IL-6 secreted by astrocytes and acting locally on other cells and structures in a carotid artery occlusion model.

To analyze the potentially detrimental effects of paracrine IL-6, it was verified that the mice did not show ischemic or white matter lesions in MRI scans within three weeks after the occlusion. Several tests were performed during the pre- and post-occlusion periods to investigate the recovery of the mice in behavioral studies. In the IL-6 overexpressing mice, there was no alteration in sickness score (modified de Simoni's neuroscore, $p=0.15$) or fine and gross-motor skills assessed by staircase pellet reaching (right paw: $p=0.64$, left paw: $p=0.74$) and RotaRod ($p=0.34$) up to 21 days after surgery (all tests 2-way ANOVA with Sidak's multiple comparison test, *Publication 1, Figure 2*). This confirmed that moderate increases of IL-6 do not exhibit negative effects in a CCA occlusion setting.

Looking at connectivity within different brain regions, significant changes were detected in 17 out of 23562 connections when the threshold was $p<0.001$. Out of these, 14 were verified as existing connections by cross-checking in tracing databases. Overall, more connections increased (10) than reduced (4) in connectivity. While intra- and inter-hemispheric connectivity increased mainly in the basal ganglia and the axis from the contralateral motor cortex to the ipsilateral pallidum, reduced connectivity remained intra-hemispheric (*Publication 1, Figure 3*). This qualitative analysis of network remodeling indicates a possible gain of function on the contralateral side to compensate for minor losses on the ipsilateral side.

The next step was to analyze the molecular changes caused by paracrine IL-6 to pinpoint potential mediators of the observed remodeling or other possibly beneficial factors in CCA occlusion. To this end, tissue was sampled from ipsilateral striatal fiber tracts and the contralateral motor cortex by laser capture microdissection. Both experiments showed differentially expressed proteins when a cut-off of $p<0.05$ and a false discovery rate (FDR) of 1 % were set. Several possibly harmful molecules such as synuclein-gamma and proenkephalin, both associated with degenerative processes, [49,50] as well as proteins that may exert neuroplastic abilities, such as caprin-1 and protein phosphatase 1 regulatory subunit 1A, where detected with high abundance in the striatal samples.[51,52] In total, 16 out of 2075 detected proteins had altered expression. The cortical samples showed 13 out of 2578 differentially expressed proteins. Most of them were membrane- or transport-associated, suggesting a role in fine-tuning neuronal vesicle transport. One example is the downregulation of Slc6a1, also known as Gat1, a γ-aminobutyric acid (GABA) transporter in the synaptic cleft. Caprin-1 and Gat1 regulation – among the most strongly altered hits for the striatum or cortex, respectively – were verified by immunohistochemical staining.

3.2 SorCS2 is secreted by astrocytes and regulates endostatin after stroke

In the second study, the main results comprise the discovery of SorCS2 upregulation in astrocytes after stroke and the analysis of its role in the physiological and post-stroke situation in mice.[53]

SorCS2 expression, until now only shown in neurons, is induced in astrocytes in an ischemic stroke mouse model and stroke patients (*Publication 2, Figure1*). This is especially the case for the glial scar region, the peri-infarct area, and parts of the contralateral cortex.

Transforming growth factor beta 1 (TGF-β1) is a cytokine associated with stroke recovery processes, most notably angiogenesis.[54,55] Its expression is upregulated after stroke in patients and mice.[56,57] TGF-β1 was also upregulated in the ischemic hemisphere in this study. This led to an upregulation of SorCS2 mRNA in primary murine and human astrocyte cultures and increased SorCS2 protein in the murine cells (*Publication 2, Figure 2*). This effect of TGF-β1 was not seen in primary neurons.

SorCS2 knock-out mice had comparable lesion sizes and astrocytic activation seen by GFAP-measured astrogliosis (*Publication 2, Figure 3*) on day three after MCAo. A measured cytokine panel of 24 cytokines showed no differential expression between SorCS2 deficient mice and controls or hemispheres for 11 proteins, mainly interleukins and interferon gamma (IFNγ) (*Publication 2, Figure S5*). Remarkably, this was also true for IL-6, which we hypothesized to be regulated by SorCS2. Other cytokines were regulated between hemispheres but not between experimental groups.

A protein array of brain tissue samples was used to identify specific proteins regulated by SorCS2 by comparing wild-type and knock-out mice. Two target proteins, insulin-like growth factor-binding protein 3 (IGFBP3) and endostatin, were not induced to the same degree as in control mice (*Publication 2, Figure 4a - c*). The focus was on endostatin as it exhibits anti-angiogenic effects and is a protein of interest in other post-stroke studies acting via modulation of the mitogen activated protein kinase (MAPK/ERK) signaling pathway.[16,58,59] Endostatin levels correlated to the size of the ischemic lesion and remained brain exclusive in wild-type mice. The lack of endostatin upregulation and increased ERK phosphorylation on the ipsilateral hemisphere was confirmed in SorCS2-deficient mice. (*Publication 2, Figure 4d – g and Figure S7*).

To support the *in vivo* results, experiments with primary astrocytic cells in culture with stimulated cytokine production using phorbol 12-myristate 13-acetate (PMA) and ionomycin. In line with previous findings, SorCS2 knock-out mice had a reduced expression and cell levels of endostatin while secreting other cytokines normally (*Publication 2, Figure 5*). Transcript levels of the endostatin precursor collagen XVIII were identical to controls, suggesting regulation of proteolysis of collagen XVIII or other post-translational mechanisms. This further proved that astrocytes secrete endostatin in a SorCS2-dependent manner.

Looking at the effects of SorCS2, modulation of angiogenesis seems likely. Investigation of vessels 21 days after MCAo with DyLight488-labeled lectin showed an increase in vessel area and length in the ipsilateral brain half in wild-type mice, especially in the glial scar region and the peri-infarct area, , while the contralateral side remained unchanged. There was no increase in SorCS2-deficient mice, independent of the hemisphere (*Publication 2, Figure 6 and S9*).

In summary, the study shows for the first time that SorCS2 is upregulated in astrocytes after ischemic stroke, exhibiting effects on the expression of endostatin and angiogenesis.

3.3 A data driven approach using machine learning provides humane endpoints in murine stroke models

The third study reviews current methods for the determination of humane endpoints and provides novel models for endpoint prediction in murine sepsis and stroke models.[47] My contribution focused on the stroke model and the data evaluation, so I will exclusively highlight the results of this part.

Initially, we wanted to assess the effects of local and systemic IL-6 in the brain. Similar to the astrocytic mouse model, we could induce IL-6 systemically with low tamoxifen doses in the endothelial FLEX-IL6 mouse model. Amounts of 40 mg/kg body weight on one to three consecutive days led to a positive feedback loop of IL-6, resulting in a cytokine storm and ultimately to a SIRS-like state of the mice with severe sickness behavior. Mice had to be euthanized at a specific sickness state or even died before a humane endpoint could be set, so that behavioral studies were not possible. This led to the question whether we could predict if an animal will die in an experiment based on body measurements and behavioral data. Subsequently, we standardized the selection of behavioral tests and time points and compiled the existing data into one coherent data set that allows for secondary use of the data.

The data for training the models were selected and compiled from a multitude of behavioral experiments in which MCAo was studied for 21 days. Sham-operated animals served as controls. Parameters monitored include daily weight and core body temperature and a modified DeSimoni's neuroscore as a sickness indicator on day -5 before and day 1, 2, 7, 14, and 21 after ischemia. The score ranges from 0, indicating no impairment, to 42, maximum impairment.

When comparing data, there was a drop in body temperature in MCAo mice during the first 5 days after surgery compared to baseline values. For non-surviving animals, this decrease is 3.5 °C higher than for surviving animals. The weight decreased in all groups, again most prominently in the non-survivor group, where the average weight loss was 5.9 g compared to 4 g in survivors and 2.4 g in controls. Neuroscores on days 1 and 2 after MCAo compared to baseline were again lowest in sham animals (4), prominent in MCAo survivors (8.77), and highest in non-survivors (15) (*Publication 3, Table 3A*). Generally, the highest scores were observed on day 1 after surgery.

All data were gathered, and two sets of parameters used for training: the values of the measurements and the change per time-point of the values with subtraction of the baseline value. Parameters considered for analysis were time points before the average time of death after MCAo (3.9 days). As the weight differed significantly between genders (p <0.001, Mann-Whitney U test), both genders were analyzed separately.

Prediction models based on Gaussian Naïve Bayes set boundaries using a single parameter were able to correctly predict death with an accuracy of 90.7 % for male mice and 86.3 % in female mice, when using only the weight change on day 3 or 2 in females, respectively. Accuracy, sensitivity, and precision were further improved when other parameters were added. For males, a combination of weight change on days 1 and 3 and the core body temperature as parameters for the model yielded an accuracy of 93.2 %. Using this prediction model, 13 out of 23 animals could have been euthanized one day earlier on day 3, while the average time to death was 4.08 days after surgery. In female mice, the best parameter combination was neuroscore, weight change, and core temperature change on day 2. With this model, 4 out of 10 animals could have been euthanized earlier on day 2, while the average time to death was 4.25 days after surgery.

3 out of 77 animals (3.95 %) were wrongly predicted to die by the algorithm and survived in the experiment (*Publication 3, Figure 2A, B and Table 4A*).

4. Discussion

This thesis unravels the molecular and structural impact of two signaling molecules on the ischemic brain periphery during recovery. Consequently, it presents novel targets for new therapeutic options in carotid artery occlusion and ischemic stroke. This thesis

(1) analyzed the effects of brain exclusive IL-6 increase in unilateral carotid occlusion in mice and found an increase in brain connectivity for 10 out of 14 altered connections and presented Caprin-1 and Gat1 as potential therapeutic targets out of 39 differentially expressed proteins in the local proteome.

(2) investigated the role of SorCS2 in post-stroke angiogenesis and recovery, showed novel expression of SorCS2 by reactive astrocytes, and found a link between SorCS2 and endostatin expression.

(3) contributed to the re-use of data and reduction of animal suffering in experimental research by aggregating data into one cohesive dataset and training an algorithm to find humane endpoints in animal models.

4.1 Summary, interpretation and embedding into the state of the art research

The first study shows that IL-6 does not lead to detrimental effects in a moderate recovery period but instead fosters the formation of intra- and inter-hemispheric connections. Additionally, it leads to the differential expression of several proteins relevant to brain regeneration and cognitive function retention. We demonstrate that brain-exclusive paracrine-acting IL-6 alone does not cause obvious behavioral deficits in the assessment of fine and gross motor skills and the overall health status. In carotid stenosis patients, IL-6 levels are usually measured only in the blood and not in the brain. High blood IL-6 levels are a poor prognostic marker and are a characteristic of unstable plaques and thus affecting patients' health.[36,37]. Elevated systemic IL-6 levels might influence the health status in CCAo mice but are not studied in this thesis due to the dosage difficulties in the VECdh-Cre-ERT2; FLEX-IL6 mouse model.

Using connectome analysis, we found that connectivity increase outweighs decreases in this paracrine IL-6 model. This is especially true between the hemispheres and in the hindbrain, particularly in the periaqueductal grey. This region serves as a relay between the brainstem and the forebrain, suggesting a stronger motor signaling towards the spinal cord.[60]

In the subsequent proteome analysis, we identified differentially regulated candidates that present attractive targets for modulating regeneration and preventing the loss of cerebral function. Possible detrimental and beneficial effects through up- or downregulation of specific proteins were found in both analyzed regions. We selected the most interesting targets for a potential intervention based on the strongest regulation and the effects reported in previous studies and confirmed them in using immunohistology: Caprin-1 and Gat1. Caprin-1 upregulation is associated with the formation of stress granules.[61] It plays a role in establishing long-term potentiation (LTP) and might be necessary for regenerative plasticity.[51] The widely downregulated protein Gat1 is an axonal transporter, removing GABA from the synaptic cleft and negatively regulating GABA-signaling.[62] This regulation is exciting, as specifically the GABAergic axis from the ipsilateral dorsal thalamic nuclei to the ipsilateral pallidum and contralateral motor area was increased in DTI analysis. This indicates an even more pronounced strengthening of GABA signaling between the thalamus and motor cortex. Higher GABA levels in this circuit were associated with less severe symptoms in Parkinson's patients.[63] In contrast, GABAergic signaling is critical for the long-term inhibition of synaptic transmission.[64] Full removal of Gat1 was shown to cause learning deficits, while Gat1 reduction led to improved learning, indicating the need for specific dosing to achieve beneficial effects.[65,66] Tiagabine, a Gat1 inhibitor drug, is used to treat epilepsy patients without impairing cognitive function.[67] In the acutely ischemic brain, tiagabine treatment showed neuroprotective effects.[68,69] Further analysis of the impact of Gat1-inhibition by tiagabine in carotid occlusion will yield attractive options in an alternative ischemic setting. The same is true for following up on other hits like the lower expression protein Vamp3, shown to limit microglial activity after surgical trauma, or high expression Atpif1, able to rescue cells in hypoxia.[70,71] Studying these molecules is more challenging with regard to the subsequent translation into the clinic, as no established treatment option is readily available.

In the second study, we unraveled that reactive astrocytes express SorCS2 after stroke. Until now, expression was only confirmed by neuronal cells.[42] The activation of expression is likely mediated by TGF-β1, validated by astrocyte culture experiments. Effects of abolishing SorCS2 were no induction of endostatin expression. Control mice had a notable endostatin increase after MCAo. SorCS2 depletion did not affect lesion size or cytokine expression, indicating a particular role in post-stroke modulation. This was surprising as it disproved that IL-6 secretion is mediated by SorCS2 receptor sorting and of the VPS10p receptors, only SorLA is responsible for IL-6 shuttling.[45] Most likely, SorCS2 modulates the post-ischemic micromilieu by affecting angiogenesis via endostatin levels, regulating the conversion from its precursor collagen XVIII. Endostatin inhibits angiogenesis in tumor models and can reverse pro-angiogenetic effects of physical activity after MCAo in mice.[16] 21 days post-stroke, we found that SorCS2 knock-out mice had reduced vessel counts in the ischemic hemisphere, which seems to contradict the accompanying lowered endostatin levels. Angiogenesis, especially after stroke, is an orchestrated and timed process triggered by a balance of pro- and anti-angiogenic molecules activated by hypoxia.[72,73] A general boost of new vessel formation by VEGF has, for example, improved and complicated post-stroke regeneration due to the leaky nature of the newly formed vessels, which are prone to edema-formation. At the same time, angiopoietin co-release helps mitigate the leakiness.[74] This highlights the complex role of post-stroke angiogenesis, where SorCS2 is a decisive factor, as shown by this study

The third study provides a systematic overview of current approaches to reduce animal suffering by determining humane endpoints in various disease models and provides machine-learning based tools to reliably identify animals that can be spared additional suffering in stroke and sepsis models. In preparation for the study, all research protocols for behavioral experiments in stroke models were standardized, data collection unified, and one extensive database generated. This allowed the development of the machine learning algorithm on a large set of experimental data with extremely high sample sizes and thus a high statistical power. Humane endpoints in murine stroke models were not assessed previously to this study. There are several other studies on humane endpoints in animal research in different disease models as explicitly listed in this publication.[47] Due to the high specificity of the mouse models, the algorithms cannot be transferred to other mouse models. Another benefit of the presented prediction model is the use of common measurements such as core body temperature, weight changes, and neuroscore. These cause no additional handling stress for the animals. Assessing whether an animal has reached the humane endpoint can be easily integrated into the ongoing research based on measurements recorded daily. The standardization of research protocols will allow a growing pool of research data and potentially expand meta-research approaches.

4.2 Strengths and weaknesses

The first study investigates the effects of paracrine-acting IL-6 in a unilateral carotid occlusion model to explore global changes in connectivity and therapeutic targets with a more distinct mechanism of action than IL-6. This investigative approach leaves room for more in-depth studies. It does not provide a complete insight into the mechanisms of IL-6 signaling in the model used, which is also reflected in the sample size. Besides, similar unilateral CCAo rodent models have caused spatial memory and object recognition impairments, accompanied by elevated IL-6 levels.[75,76] The study shows connectivity changes involving motor fibers but with no apparent effects on motor behavior. This could be attributable to the low sensitivity of the behavioral tests and the relatively subtle effects of altered brain connections. Long-term follow-up and further behavioral studies, including memory testing, can help unravel the potential of IL-6 in CCAo even more.

Using LCM to isolate fiber tracts is a promising technique. Previously, proteome analysis of fiber tracts was only successful in the developing mouse or using advanced methods due to high-fat content of the tissue.[77,78]

The model for astrocytic IL-6 activation does lead to a permanent secretion of IL-6, even though levels remain moderate and confined to the brain. IL-6 is a cytokine with various effects, and thus, we cannot exclude that this might cause more detrimental effects in the long term. Therefore, we focused on finding proteins serving as potential targets rather than trying to unravel detailed dose- and time-dependent short- and long-term consequences.

The SorCS2 study stresses the importance of anti-angiogenic proteins in post-stroke recovery and provides novel insights about SorCS2 after stroke, especially its secretion by astrocytes. This study used a constitutive knock-out model, and it cannot be excluded that the effects of neuronal SorCS2 outweigh and even compensate for the lack of astrocytic SorCS2. Further studies with a conditional knock-out at the time of injury or shortly after can address this and provide a better insight into the specific post-stroke effects of the sortilin receptor. As mentioned above, angiogenesis is a complex process, and we focused on SorCS2 alone. More detailed insights will be possible with further studies analyzing the interplay between relevant mediators of angiogenesis such as VEGF and SorCS2.

The presented algorithms provide a simple tool to prevent unnecessary suffering in commonly used animal models in behavioral research. However, 24 – 36 h is a relatively short period of time to reduce suffering. As the data set is comparatively small for a machine learning approach, especially in the non-survivor group, further optimization can be achieved by continuously updating the model or using more data, for example, continuous measurement of body temperature. The novel database is a valuable resource for new approaches in animal research using meta-research. Larger sample sizes allow better-powered analyses without further inflicting damage to animals and are a starting point to generate and test hypotheses without the need for new behavioral studies.

Melanie Tamara Carolin Kuffner
Mechanisms of Adaptation and Reconstruction in the Hypoperfused Brain

5. Conclusions

This thesis investigates the astrocyte-mediated molecular adaptations after focal ischemia and carotid occlusion by evaluating the effects of IL-6 and SorCS2. Both mediated beneficial effects in our study settings. Due to the complex interplay both molecules have the potential to negatively affect outcomes in different disease models or in the long term. Contrary to the initial hypothesis, we did not find a direct link between both molecules.

The unified data gathered from murine stroke models allowed to build a large database with physiological and behavioral data. This was the prerequisite to developing an algorithm that predicts humane endpoints and can prevent animal suffering in future behavioral tests with murine MCAo models. It also gives the opportunity to answer future research question using existing data and reduces the need for animals in research. This thesis conducts preclinical research and provides the target molecules Caprin-1, Gat1, SorCS2 and endostatin. After verification in preclinical and clinical studies, these molecules and are exciting options for the treatment of stroke and carotid stenosis.

Reference List

1. Statistisches Bundesamt (Destatis). Causes of death by chapters of the ICD-10 and gender. https://www.destatis.de/EN/Themes/Society-Environment/Health/Causes-Death/Tables/number-of-death.html (2021).

2. Heron, M. Deaths: leading causes for 2019. *National Vital Statistics Reports* **70**, 1–113 (2021).

3. Johnson, C. O., Roth, G. A., Bisignano, C., Abady, G. G., Abbasifard, M., Abbasi-Kangevari, M., Abd-Allah, F., Abedi, V., Abualhasan, A., Abu-Rmeileh, N. M., Abushouk, A. I., Adebayo, O. M., Agarwal, G., Agasthi, P., Ahinkorah, B. O., Ahmad, S., Ahmadi, S., Salih, Y. A., Aji, B., Akbarpour, S., Akinyemi, R. O., Hamad, H. al, Alahdab, F., Alif, S. M., Alipour, V., Aljunid, S. M., Almustanyir, S., Al-Raddadi, R. M., Salman, R. A.-S., Alvis-Guzman, N., Ancuceanu, R., Anderlini, D., Anderson, J. A., Ansar, A., Antonazzo, I. C., Arabloo, J., Ärnlöv, J., Artanti, K. D., Aryan, Z., Asgari, S., Ashraf, T., Athar, M., Atreya, A., Ausloos, M., Baig, A. A., Baltatu, O. C., Banach, M., Barboza, M. A., Barker-Collo, S. L., Bärnighausen, T. W., Barone, M. T. U., Basu, S., Bazmandegan, G., Beghi, E., Beheshti, M., Béjot, Y., Bell, A. W., Bennett, D. A., Bensenor, I. M., Bezabhe, W. M., Bezabih, Y. M., Bhagavathula, A. S., Bhardwaj, P., Bhattacharyya, K., Bijani, A., Bikbov, B., Birhanu, M. M., Boloor, A., Bonny, A., Brauer, M., Brenner, H., Bryazka, D., Butt, Z. A., Santos, F. L. C. dos, Campos-Nonato, I. R., Cantu-Brito, C., Carrero, J. J., Castañeda-Orjuela, C. A., Catapano, A. L., Chakraborty, P. A., Charan, J.,

Choudhari, S. G., Chowdhury, E. K., Chu, D.-T., Chung, S.-C., Colozza, D., Costa, V. M., Costanzo, S., Criqui, M. H., Dadras, O., Dagnew, B., Dai, X., Dalal, K., Damasceno, A. A. M., D'Amico, E., Dandona, L., Dandona, R., Gela, J. D., Davletov, K., Cruz-Góngora, V. D. la, Desai, R., Dhamnetiya, D., Dharmaratne, S. D., Dhimal, M. L., Dhimal, M., Diaz, D., Dichgans, M., Dokova, K., Doshi, R., Douiri, A., Duncan, B. B., Eftekharzadeh, S., Ekholuenetale, M., Nahas, N. el, Elgendy, I. Y., Elhadi, M., El-Jaafary, S. I., Endres, M., Endries, A. Y., Erku, D. A., Faraon, E. J. A., Farooque, U., Farzadfar, F., Feroze, A. H., Filip, I., Fischer, F., Flood, D., Gad, M. M., Gaidhane, S., Gheshlagh, R. G., Ghashghaee, A., Ghith, N., Ghozali, G., Ghozy, S., Gialluisi, A., Giampaoli, S., Gilani, S. A., Gill, P. S., Gnedovskaya, E. v, Golechha, M., Goulart, A. C., Guo, Y., Gupta, R., Gupta, V. B., Gupta, V. K., Gyanwali, P., Hafezi-Nejad, N., Hamidi, S., Hanif, A., Hankey, G. J., Hargono, A., Hashi, A., Hassan, T. S., Hassen, H. Y., Havmoeller, R. J., Hay, S. I., Hayat, K., Hegazy, M. I., Herteliu, C., Holla, R., Hostiuc, S., Househ, M., Huang, J., Humayun, A., Hwang, B.-F., Iacoviello, L., Iavicoli, I., Ibitoye, S. E., Ilesanmi, O. S., Ilic, I. M., Ilic, M. D., Iqbal, U., Irvani, S. S. N., Islam, S. M. S., Ismail, N. E., Iso, H., Isola, G., Iwagami, M., Jacob, L., Jain, V., Jang, S.-I., Jayapal, S. K., Jayaram, S., Jayawardena, R., Jeemon, P., Jha, R. P., Johnson, W. D., Jonas, J. B., Joseph, N., Jozwiak, J. J., Jürisson, M., Kalani, R., Kalhor, R., Kalkonde, Y., Kamath, A., Kamiab, Z., Kanchan, T., Kandel, H., Karch, A., Katoto, P. D., Kayode, G. A., Keshavarz, P., Khader, Y. S., Khan, E. A., Khan, I. A., Khan, M., Khan, M. A., Khatib, M. N., Khubchandani, J., Kim, G. R., Kim, M. S., Kim, Y. J., Kisa, A., Kisa, S., Kivimäki, M., Kolte, D., Koolivand, A., Laxminarayana, S. L. K., Koyanagi, A., Krishan,

K., Krishnamoorthy, V., Krishnamurthi, R. v, Kumar, G. A., Kusuma, D., Vecchia, C. la, Lacey, B., Lak, H. M., Lallukka, T., Lasrado, S., Lavados, P. M., Leonardi, M., Li, B., Li, S., Lin, H., Lin, R.-T., Liu, X., Lo, W. D., Lorkowski, S., Lucchetti, G., Saute, R. L., Razek, H. M. A. el, Magnani, F. G., Mahajan, P. B., Majeed, A., Makki, A., Malekzadeh, R., Malik, A. A., Manafi, N., Mansournia, M. A., Mantovani, L. G., Martini, S., Mazzaglia, G., Mehndiratta, M. M., Menezes, R. G., Meretoja, A., Mersha, A. G., Jonasson, J. M., Miazgowski, B., Miazgowski, T., Michalek, I. M., Mirrakhimov, E. M., Mohammad, Y., Mohammadian-Hafshejani, A., Mohammed, S., Mokdad, A. H., Mokhayeri, Y., Molokhia, M., Moni, M. A., Montasir, A. al, Moradzadeh, R., Morawska, L., Morze, J., Muruet, W., Musa, K. I., Nagarajan, A. J., Naghavi, M., Swamy, S. N., Nascimento, B. R., Negoi, R. I., Kandel, S. N., Nguyen, T. H., Norrving, B., Noubiap, J. J., Nwatah, V. E., Oancea, B., Odukoya, O. O., Olagunju, A. T., Orru, H., Owolabi, M. O., Padubidri, J. R., Pana, A., Parekh, T., Park, E.-C., Kan, F. P., Pathak, M., Peres, M. F. P., Perianayagam, A., Pham, T.-M., Piradov, M. A., Podder, V., Polinder, S., Postma, M. J., Pourshams, A., Radfar, A., Rafiei, A., Raggi, A., Rahim, F., Rahimi-Movaghar, V., Rahman, M., Rahman, M. A., Rahmani, A. M., Rajai, N., Ranasinghe, P., Rao, C. R., Rao, S. J., Rathi, P., Rawaf, D. L., Rawaf, S., Reitsma, M. B., Renjith, V., Renzaho, A. M. N., Rezapour, A., Rodriguez, J. A. B., Roever, L., Romoli, M., Rynkiewicz, A., Sacco, S., Sadeghi, M., Moghaddam, S. S., Sahebkar, A., Saif-Ur-Rahman, K., Salah, R., Samaei, M., Samy, A. M., Santos, I. S., Santric-Milicevic, M. M., Sarrafzadegan, N., Sathian, B., Sattin, D., Schiavolin, S., Schlaich, M. P., Schmidt, M. I., Schutte, A. E., Sepanlou, S. G., Seylani, A., Sha, F., Shahabi,

S., Shaikh, M. A., Shannawaz, M., Shawon, M. S. R., Sheikh, A., Sheikhbahaei, S., Shibuya, K., Siabani, S., Silva, D. A. S., Singh, J. A., Singh, J. K., Skryabin, V. Y., Skryabina, A. A., Sobaih, B. H., Stortecky, S., Stranges, S., Tadesse, E. G., Tarigan, I. U., Temsah, M.-H., Teuschl, Y., Thrift, A. G., Tonelli, M., Tovani-Palone, M. R., Tran, B. X., Tripathi, M., Tsegaye, G. W., Ullah, A., Unim, B., Unnikrishnan, B., Vakilian, A., Tahbaz, S. V., Vasankari, T. J., Venketasubramanian, N., Vervoort, D., Vo, B., Volovici, V., Vosoughi, K., Vu, G. T., Vu, L. G., Wafa, H. A., Waheed, Y., Wang, Y., Wijeratne, T., Winkler, A. S., Wolfe, C. D. A., Woodward, M., Wu, J. H., Hanson, S. W., Xu, X., Yadav, L., Yadollahpour, A., Jabbari, S. H. Y., Yamagishi, K., Yatsuya, H., Yonemoto, N., Yu, C., Yunusa, I., Zaman, M. S., Zaman, S. bin, Zamanian, M., Zand, R., Zandifar, A., Zastrozhin, M. S., Zastrozhina, A., Zhang, Y., Zhang, Z.-J., Zhong, C., Zuniga, Y. M. H. & Murray, C. J. L. Global, regional, and national burden of stroke and its risk factors, 1990-2019: a systematic analysis for the Global Burden of Disease Study 2019. *The Lancet Neurology* **20**, 795–820 (2021).

4. Fieschi, C., Argentino, C., Lenzi, G. L., Sacchetti, M. L., Toni, D. & Bozzao, L. Clinical and instrumental evaluation of patients with ischemic stroke within the first six hours. *J Neurol Sci* **91**, 311–321 (1989).

5. Lal, B. K., Dux, M. C., Sikdar, S., Goldstein, C., Khan, A. A., Yokemick, J. & Zhao, L. Asymptomatic carotid stenosis is associated with cognitive impairment. *Journal of Vascular Surgery* **66**, 1083–1092 (2017).

6. de Los Ríos la Rosa, F., Khoury, J., Kissela, B. M., Flaherty, M. L., Alwell, K., Moomaw, C. J., Khatri, P., Adeoye, O., Woo, D., Ferioli, S. & Kleindorfer, D. O. Eligibility for Intravenous Recombinant Tissue-Type Plasminogen Activator Within a Population The Effect of the European Cooperative Acute Stroke Study (ECASS) III Trial. *Stroke* **43**, 1591–1595 (2012).

7. Yang, P., Zhang, Y., Zhang, L., Zhang, Y., Treurniet, K. M., Chen, W., Peng, Y., Han, H., Wang, J., Wang, S., Yin, C., Liu, S., Wang, P., Fang, Q., Shi, H., Yang, J., Wen, C., Li, C., Jiang, C., Sun, J., Yue, X., Lou, M., Zhang, M., Shu, H., Sun, D., Liang, H., Li, T., Guo, F., Ke, K., Yuan, H., Wang, G., Yang, W., Shi, H., Li, T., Li, Z., Xing, P., Zhang, P., Zhou, Y., Wang, H., Xu, Y., Huang, Q., Wu, T., Zhao, R., Li, Q., Fang, Y., Wang, L., Lu, J., Li, Y., Fu, J., Zhong, X., Wang, Y., Wang, L., Goyal, M., Dippel, D. W. J., Hong, B., Deng, B., Roos, Y. B. W. E. M., Majoie, C. B. L. M. & Liu, J. Endovascular Thrombectomy with or without Intravenous Alteplase in Acute Stroke. *New England Journal of Medicine* **382**, 1981–1993 (2020).

8. Casetta, I., Fainardi, E., Saia, V., Pracucci, G., Padroni, M., Renieri, L., Nencini, P., Inzitari, D., Morosetti, D., Sallustio, F., Vallone, S., Bigliardi, G., Zini, A., Longo, M., Francalanza, I., Bracco, S., Vallone, I. M., Tassi, R., Bergui, M., Naldi, A., Saletti, A., de Vito, A., Gasparotti, R., Magoni, M., Castellan, L., Castellan, L., Serrati, C., Menozzi, R., Scoditti, U., Causin, F., Pieroni, A., Puglielli, E., Casalena, A., Sanna, A., Ruggiero, M., Cordici, F., di Maggio, L., Duc, E., Cosottini, M., Giannini, N., Sanfilippo, G., Zappoli, F., Toni, D., Cavasin, N., Critelli, A., Ciceri, E., Plebani, M., Cappellari, M., Chiumarulo, L., Petruzzellis, M.,

Terrana, A., Cariddi, L. P., Burdi, N., Tinelli, A., Auteri, W., Silvagni, U., Biraschi, F., Nicolini, E., Padolecchia, R., Tassinari, T., Filauri, P., Sacco, S., Pavia, M., Invernizzi, P., Nuzzi, N. P., Marcheselli, S., Amistà, P., Russo, M., Gallesio, I., Gallesio, I., Craparo, G., Mannino, M. & Mangiafico, S. Endovascular Thrombectomy for Acute Ischemic Stroke Beyond 6 Hours From Onset: A Real-World Experience. *Stroke* **51**, 2051–2057 (2020).

9. Brouns, R. & De Deyn, P. P. The complexity of neurobiological processes in acute ischemic stroke. *Clinical Neurology and Neurosurgery* **111**, 483–495 (2009).

10. Wakita, H., Tomimoto, H., Akiguchi, I. & Kimura, J. Glial activation and white matter changes in the rat brain induced by chronic cerebral hypoperfusion: an immunohistochemical study. *Acta Neuropathologica* **87**, 484–492 (1994).

11. Ueno, M., Nakamura, Y., Li, J., Goulding, M., Baccei, M. L., Ueno, M., Nakamura, Y., Li, J., Gu, Z., Niehaus, J., Maezawa, M. & Crone, S. A. Corticospinal Circuits from the Sensory and Motor Cortices Differentially Regulate Skilled Movements through Distinct Spinal Interneurons Article Corticospinal Circuits from the Sensory and Motor Cortices Differentially Regulate Skilled Movements through Distinct Spinal Interneurons. *CellReports* **23**, 1286-1300.e7 (2018).

12. Holland, P. R., Searcy, J. L., Salvadores, N., Scullion, G., Chen, G., Lawson, G., Scott, F., Bastin, M. E., Ihara, M., Kalaria, R., Wood, E. R., Smith, C., Wardlaw, J. M. & Horsburgh, K. Gliovascular disruption and cognitive deficits in a mouse model with

features of small vessel disease. *J Cereb Blood Flow Metab* **35**, 1005–1014 (2015).

13. Duncombe, J., Kitamura, A., Hase, Y., Ihara, M., Kalaria, R. N. & Horsburgh, K. Chronic cerebral hypoperfusion: A key mechanism leading to vascular cognitive impairment and dementia. Closing the translational gap between rodent models and human vascular cognitive impairment and dementia. *Clinical Science* **131**, 2451–2468 (2017).

14. Bachmann, L. C., Lindau, N. T., Felder, P. & Schwab, M. E. Sprouting of brainstem-spinal tracts in response to unilateral motor cortex stroke in mice. *J Neurosci* **34**, 3378–3389 (2014).

15. Hoffmann, C. J., Harms, U., Rex, A., Szulzewsky, F., Wolf, S. A., Grittner, U., Lättig-Tünnemann, G., Sendtner, M., Kettenmann, H., Dirnagl, U., Endres, M. & Harms, C. Vascular signal transducer and activator of transcription-3 promotes angiogenesis and neuroplasticity long-term after stroke. *Circulation* **131**, 1772–1782 (2015).

16. Gertz, K., Priller, J., Kronenberg, G., Fink, K. B., Winter, B., Schröck, H., Ji, S., Milosevic, M., Harms, C., Böhm, M., Dirnagl, U., Laufs, U. & Endres, M. Physical activity improves long-term stroke outcome via endothelial nitric oxide synthase-dependent augmentation of neovascularization and cerebral blood flow. *Circulation Research* **99**, 1132–1140 (2006).

17. Hermann, D. M. & Zechariah, A. Implications of vascular endothelial growth factor for postischemic neurovascular remodeling. *J Cereb Blood Flow Metab* **29**, 1620–1643 (2009).

18. Snapyan, M., Lemasson, M., Brill, M. S., Blais, M., Massouh, M., Ninkovic, J., Gravel, C., Berthod, F., Götz, M., Barker, P. A., Parent, A. & Saghatelyan, A. Vasculature guides migrating neuronal precursors in the adult mammalian forebrain via brain-derived neurotrophic factor signaling. *J Neurosci* **29**, 4172–4188 (2009).

19. Anrather, J. & Iadecola, C. Inflammation and Stroke: An Overview. *Neurotherapeutics* **13**, 661–670 (2016).

20. Beck, H. & Plate, K. H. Angiogenesis after cerebral ischemia. *Acta Neuropathologica* **117**, 481–496 (2009).

21. Nishihiro, S., Hishikawa, T., Hiramatsu, M., Kidani, N., Takahashi, Y., Murai, S., Sugiu, K., Higaki, Y., Yasuhara, T., Borlongan, C. V. & Date, I. High-Mobility Group Box-1-Induced Angiogenesis After Indirect Bypass Surgery in a Chronic Cerebral Hypoperfusion Model. *NeuroMolecular Medicine* **21**, 391–400 (2019).

22. Zhang, W., Petrovic, J. M., Callaghan, D., Jones, A., Cui, H., Howlett, C. & Stanimirovic, D. Evidence that hypoxia-inducible factor-1 (HIF-1) mediates transcriptional activation of interleukin-1beta (IL-1beta) in astrocyte cultures. *J Neuroimmunol* **174**, 63–73 (2006).

23. Liu, Q., Bhuiyan, M. I. H., Liu, R., Song, S., Begum, G., Young, C. B., Foley, L. M., Chen, F., Hitchens, T. K., Cao, G., Chattopadhyay, A., He, L. & Sun, D. Attenuating vascular stenosis-induced astrogliosis preserves white matter integrity and cognitive function. *Journal of Neuroinflammation* **18**, 187 (2021).

24. Ito, M., Komai, K., Mise-Omata, S., Iizuka-Koga, M., Noguchi, Y., Kondo, T., Sakai, R., Matsuo, K., Nakayama, T., Yoshie, O., Nakatsukasa, H., Chikuma, S., Shichita, T. & Yoshimura, A. Brain regulatory T cells suppress astrogliosis and potentiate neurological recovery. *Nature* **565**, 246–250 (2019).

25. Klein, M. A., Möller, J. C., Jones, L. L., Bluethmann, H., Kreutzberg, G. W. & Raivich, G. Impaired Neuroglial Activation in Interleukin-6 Deficient Mice. *GLIA* **19**, 227–233 (1997).

26. Balasingam, V., Tejada-Berges, T., Wright, E., Bouckova, R. & Yong, V. W. Reactive astrogliosis in the neonatal mouse brain and its modulation by cytokines. *J Neurosci* **14**, 846–856 (1994).

27. Pekny, M., Pekna, M., Messing, A., Steinhäuser, C., Lee, J. M., Parpura, V., Hol, E. M., Sofroniew, M. v. & Verkhratsky, A. Astrocytes: a central element in neurological diseases. *Acta Neuropathol* **131**, 323–345 (2016).

28. Tanaka, T., Narazaki, M. & Kishimoto, T. IL-6 in inflammation, immunity, and disease. *Cold Spring Harb Perspect Biol* **6**, a016295 (2014).

29. Bluthé, R.-M., Michaud, B., Poli, V. & Dantzer, R. Role of IL-6 in cytokine-induced sickness behavior: a study with IL-6 deficient mice. *Physiology & Behavior* **70**, 367–373 (2000).

30. Asgarov, R., Sen, K. M., Meena, M., Karl, T., Gyengesi, E., Mahns, D. A., Malladi, C. S. & Münch, G. W. Characterisation of the Mouse Cerebellar Proteome in the GFAP-IL6 Model of

Chronic Neuroinflammation. *The Cerebellum* **21**, 404–424 (2021).

31. Gyengesi, E., Rangel, A., Ullah, F., Liang, H., Niedermayer, G., Asgarov, R., Venigalla, M., Gunawardena, D., Karl, T. & Münch, G. Chronic Microglial Activation in the GFAP-IL6 Mouse Contributes to Age-Dependent Cerebellar Volume Loss and Impairment in Motor Function. *Frontiers in Neuroscience* **13**, 303 (2019).

32. Yang, P., Wen, H., Ou, S., Cui, J. & Fan, D. IL-6 promotes regeneration and functional recovery after cortical spinal tract injury by reactivating intrinsic growth program of neurons and enhancing synapse formation. *Experimental Neurology* **236**, 19–27 (2012).

33. Bowen, K., Dempsey, R. & Vemuganti, R. Adult interleukin-6 knockout mice show compromised neurogenesis. *Neuroreport* **22**, 126–130 (2011).

34. Ormstad, H., Aass, H. C. D., Lund-Sørensen, N., Amthor, K. F. & Sandvik, L. Serum levels of cytokines and C-reactive protein in acute ischemic stroke patients, and their relationship to stroke lateralization, type, and infarct volume. *Journal of Neurology* **258**, 677–685 (2011).

35. Bustamante, A., Sobrino, T., Giralt, D., García-Berrocoso, T., Llombart, V., Ugarriza, I., Espadaler, M., Rodríguez, N., Sudlow, C., Castellanos, M., Smith, C. J., Rodríguez-Yánez, M., Waje-Andreassen, U., Tanne, D., Oto, J., Barber, M., Worthmann, H., Wartenberg, K. E., Becker, K. J., Chakraborty, B., Oh, S. H.,

Whiteley, W. N., Castillo, J. & Montaner, J. Prognostic value of blood interleukin-6 in the prediction of functional outcome after stroke: A systematic review and meta-analysis. *Journal of Neuroimmunology* **274**, 215–224 (2014).

36. Puz, P. & Lasek–Bal, A. Repeated measurements of serum concentrations of TNF-alpha, interleukin-6 and interleukin-10 in the evaluation of internal carotid artery stenosis progression. *Atherosclerosis* **263**, 97–103 (2017).

37. Yamagami, H., Kitagawa, K., Nagai, Y., Hougaku, H., Sakaguchi, M., Kuwabara, K., Kondo, K., Masuyama, T., Matsumoto, M. & Hori, M. Higher Levels of Interlieukin-6 Are Associated with Lower Echogenicity of Carotid Artery Plaques. *Stroke* **35**, 677–681 (2004).

38. Gertz, K., Kronenberg, G., Kälin, R. E., Baldinger, T., Werner, C., Balkaya, M., Eom, G. D., Hellmann-Regen, J., Kröber, J., Miller, K. R., Lindauer, U., Laufs, U., Dirnagl, U., Heppner, F. L. & Endres, M. Essential role of interleukin-6 in post-stroke angiogenesis. *Brain* **135**, 1964–1680 (2012).

39. Willnow, T. E., Petersen, C. M. & Nykjaer, A. VPS10P-domain receptors — regulators of neuronal viability and function. *Nature Reviews Neuroscience* **9**, 899–909 (2008).

40. Vaegter, C. B., Jansen, P., Fjorback, A. W., Glerup, S., Skeldal, S., Kjolby, M., Richner, M., Erdmann, B., Nyengaard, J. R., Tessarollo, L., Lewin, G. R., Willnow, T. E., Chao, M. v & Nykjaer, A. Sortilin associates with Trk receptors to enhance

anterograde transport and neurotrophin signaling. *Nature Neuroscience* **14**, 54–61 (2011).

41. Chen, Z. Y., Ieraci, A., Teng, H., Dall, H., Meng, C. X., Herrera, D. G., Nykjaer, A., Hempstead, B. L. & Lee, F. S. Sortilin Controls Intracellular Sorting of Brain-Derived Neurotrophic Factor to the Regulated Secretory Pathway. *Journal of Neuroscience* **25**, 6156–6166 (2005).

42. Glerup, S., Olsen, D., Vaegter, C. B., Gustafsen, C., Sjoegaard, S. S., Hermey, G., Kjolby, M., Molgaard, S., Ulrichsen, M., Boggild, S., Skeldal, S., Fjorback, A. N., Nyengaard, J. R., Jacobsen, J., Bender, D., Bjarkam, C. R., Sørensen, E. S., Füchtbauer, E. M., Eichele, G., Madsen, P., Willnow, T. E., Petersen, C. M. & Nykjaer, A. SorCS2 Regulates Dopaminergic Wiring and Is Processed into an Apoptotic Two-Chain Receptor in Peripheral Glia. *Neuron* **82**, 1074–1087 (2014).

43. Yang, J., Ma, Q., Dincheva, I., Giza, J., Jing, D., Marinic, T., Milner, T. A., Rajadhyaksha, A., Lee, F. S. & Hempstead, B. L. SorCS2 is required for social memory and trafficking of the NMDA receptor. *Molecular Psychiatry* **26**, 927–940 (2021).

44. Malik, A. R., Szydlowska, K., Nizinska, K., Asaro, A., van Vliet, E. A., Popp, O., Dittmar, G., Fritsche-Guenther, R., Kirwan, J. A., Nykjaer, A., Lukasiuk, K., Aronica, E. & Willnow, T. E. SorCS2 Controls Functional Expression of Amino Acid Transporter EAAT3 and Protects Neurons from Oxidative Stress and Epilepsy-Induced Pathology. *Cell Reports* **26**, 2792-2804.e6 (2019).

45. Larsen, J. V. & Petersen, C. M. SorLA in Interleukin-6 Signaling and Turnover. *Molecular and Cellular Biology* **37**, e00641-16 (2017).

46. Kuffner, M., Koch, S. P., Kirchner, M., Mueller, S., Lips, J., An, J., Mertins, P., Dirnagl, U., Endres, M., Boehm-Sturm, P., Harms, C. & Hoffmann, C. J. Paracrine Interleukin 6 Induces Cerebral Remodeling at Early Stages After Unilateral Common Carotid Artery Occlusion in Mice. *Front Cardiovasc Med* **8**, (2022).

47. Mei, J., Banneke, S., Lips, J., Kuffner, M. T. C., Hoffmann, C. J., Dirnagl, U., Endres, M., Harms, C. & Emmrich, J. V. Refining humane endpoints in mouse models of disease by systematic review and machine learning-based endpoint definition. *Altex* **36**, (2019).

48. Dirnagl, U. & Group, M. of the M.-S. Standard operating procedures (SOP) in experimental stroke research: SOP for middle cerebral artery occlusion in the mouse. *Nature Precedings* (2010) doi:10.1038/npre.2010.3492.2.

49. Holm, H., Nägga, K., Nilsson, E. D., Ricci, F., Melander, O., Hansson, O., Bachus, E., Fedorowski, A. & Magnusson, M. High circulating levels of midregional proenkephalin A predict vascular dementia: a population-based prospective study. *Sci Rep* **10**, 8027 (2020).

50. Brás, I. C., Dominguez-Meijide, A., Gerhardt, E., Koss, D., Lázaro, D. F., Santos, P. I., Vasili, E., Xylaki, M. & Outeiro, T. F. Synucleinopathies: Where we are and where we need to go. *J Neurochem* **153**, 433–454 (2020).

51. Nakayama, K., Ohashi, R., Shinoda, Y., Yamazaki, M., Abe, M., Fujikawa, A., Shigenobu, S., Futatsugi, A., Noda, M., Mikoshiba, K., Furuichi, T., Sakimura, K. & Shiina, N. RNG105/caprin1, an RNA granule protein for dendritic mRNA localization, is essential for long-term memory formation. *Elife* **6**, e29677 (2017).

52. Munton, R. P., Vizi, S. & Mansuy, I. M. The role of protein phosphatase-1 in the modulation of synaptic and structural plasticity. *FEBS Lett* **567**, 121–128 (2004).

53. Malik, A. R., Lips, J., Gorniak-Walas, M., Broekaart, D. W. M., Asaro, A., Kuffner, M. T. C., Hoffmann, C. J., Kikhia, M., Dopatka, M., Boehm-Sturm, P., Mueller, S., Dirnagl, U., Aronica, E., Harms, C. & Willnow, T. E. SorCS2 facilitates release of endostatin from astrocytes and controls post-stroke angiogenesis. *GLIA* **68**, (2020).

54. Pardali, E., Goumans, M. J. & ten Dijke, P. Signaling by members of the TGF-β family in vascular morphogenesis and disease. *Trends in Cell Biology* **20**, 556–567 (2010).

55. Meng, H., Song, Y., Zhu, J., Liu, Q., Lu, P., Ye, N., Zhang, Z., Pang, Y., Qi, J. & Wu, H. LRG1 promotes angiogenesis through upregulating the TGF-β1 pathway in ischemic rat brain. *Molecular Medicine Reports* **14**, 5535–5543 (2016).

56. Yan, J., Greer, J. M. & McCombe, P. A. Prolonged elevation of cytokine levels after human acute ischaemic stroke with evidence of individual variability. *Journal of Neuroimmunology* **246**, 78–84 (2012).

57. Zhang, C., Zhu, Y., Wang, S., Wei, Z. Z., Jiang, M. Q., Zhang, Y., Pan, Y., Tao, S., Li, J. & Wei, L. Temporal gene expression profiles after focal cerebral ischemia in mice. *Aging and Disease* **9**, 249–261 (2018).

58. Chen, N., Gao, R. F., Yuan, F. L. & Zhao, M. D. Recombinant human endostatin suppresses mouse osteoclast formation by inhibiting the NF-κB and MAPKs signaling pathways. *Frontiers in Pharmacology* **7**, 145 (2016).

59. Sudhakar, A., Sugimoto, H., Yang, C., Lively, J., Zeisberg, M. & Kalluri, R. Human tumstatin and human endostatin exhibit distinct antiangiogenic activities mediated by $\alpha v\beta 3$ and $\alpha 5\beta 1$ integrins. *Proceedings of the National Academy of Sciences* **100**, 4766–4771 (2003).

60. Benarroch, E. E. Periaqueductal gray: an interface for behavioral control. *Neurology* **78**, 210–217 (2012).

61. Solomon, S., Xu, Y., Wang, B., David, M. D., Schubert, P., Kennedy, D. & Schrader, J. W. Distinct Structural Features of Caprin-1 Mediate Its Interaction with G3BP-1 and Its Induction of Phosphorylation of Eukaryotic Translation Initiation Factor 2α, Entry to Cytoplasmic Stress Granules, and Selective Interaction with a Subset of mRNAs. *Molecular and Cellular Biology* **27**, 2324–2342 (2007).

62. Borden, L. A. & Caplan, M. J. GABA transporter heterogeneity: Pharmacology and cellular localization. *Neurochemistry International* **29**, 335–356 (1996).

63. van Nuland, A. J. M., den Ouden, H. E. M., Zach, H., Dirkx, M. F. M., van Asten, J. J. A., Scheenen, T. W. J., Toni, I., Cools, R. & Helmich, R. C. GABAergic changes in the thalamocortical circuit in Parkinson's disease. *Human Brain Mapping* **41**, 1017 (2020).

64. Watanabe, M., Maemura, K., Kanbara, K., Tamayama, T. & Hayasaki, H. GABA and GABA receptors in the central nervous system and other organs. *Int Rev Cytol* **213**, 1–47 (2002).

65. Shi, J., Cai, Y., Liu, G., Gong, N., Liu, Z., Xu, T., Wang, Z. & Fei, J. Enhanced learning and memory in GAT1 heterozygous mice. *Acta Biochim Biophys Sin (Shanghai)* **44**, 359–366 (2012).

66. Yang, P., Cai, G., Cai, Y., Fei, J. & Liu, G. Gamma aminobutyric acid transporter subtype 1 gene knockout mice: a new model for attention deficit/hyperactivity disorder. *Acta Biochim Biophys Sin (Shanghai)* **45**, 578–585 (2013).

67. Äikiä, M., Jutila, L., Salmenperä, T., Mervaala, E. & Kälviäinen, R. Comparison of the cognitive effects of tiagabine and carbamazepine as monotherapy in newly diagnosed adult patients with partial epilepsy: pooled analysis of two long-term, randomized, follow-up studies. *Epilepsia* **47**, 1121–1127 (2006).

68. Lie, M. E. K., Gowing, E. K., Clausen, R. P., Wellendorph, P. & Clarkson, A. N. Inhibition of GABA transporters fails to afford significant protection following focal cerebral ischemia. *J Cereb Blood Flow Metab* **38**, 166–173 (2018).

69. Yang, Y., Li, Q., Wang, C. X., Jeerakathil, T. & Shuaib, A. Dose-dependent neuroprotection with tiagabine in a focal cerebral ischemia model in rat. *Neuroreport* **11**, 2307–2311 (2000).

70. García-Bermúdez, J. & Cuezva, J. M. The ATPase Inhibitory Factor 1 (IF1): A master regulator of energy metabolism and of cell survival. *Biochim Biophys Acta* **1857**, 1167–1182 (2016).

71. Chen, Y., Sun, J. X., Chen, W. K., Wu, G. C., Wang, Y. Q., Zhu, K. Y. & Wang, J. miR-124/VAMP3 is a novel therapeutic target for mitigation of surgical trauma-induced microglial activation. *Signal Transduct Target Ther* **4**, 27 (2019).

72. Yang, Y. & Torbey, M. T. Angiogenesis and Blood-Brain Barrier Permeability in Vascular Remodeling after Stroke. *Current Neuropharmacology* **18**, 1250 (2020).

73. Hayashi, T., Noshita, N., Sugawara, T. & Chan, P. H. Temporal profile of angiogenesis and expression of related genes in the brain after ischemia. *J Cereb Blood Flow Metab* **23**, 166–180 (2003).

74. Zhang, Z. G., Zhang, L., Jiang, Q., Zhang, R., Davies, K., Powers, C., Van Bruggen, N. & Chopp, M. VEGF enhances angiogenesis and promotes blood-brain barrier leakage in the ischemic brain. *Journal of Clinical Investigation* **106**, 829 (2000).

75. Yoshizaki, K., Adachi, K., Kataoka, S., Watanabe, A., Tabira, T., Takahashi, K. & Wakita, H. Chronic cerebral hypoperfusion induced by right unilateral common carotid artery occlusion causes delayed white matter lesions and cognitive impairment in adult mice. *Experimental Neurology* **210**, 585–591 (2008).

76. Mansour, A., Niizuma, K., Rashad, S., Sumiyoshi, A., Ryoke, R., Endo, H., Endo, T., Sato, K., Kawashima, R. & Tominaga, T. A refined model of chronic cerebral hypoperfusion resulting in cognitive impairment and a low mortality rate in rats. *Journal of Neurosurgery* **131**, 892–902 (2019).

77. Fuller, H. R., Slade, R., Jovanov-Milošević, N., Babić, M., Sedmak, G., Šimić, G., Fuszard, M. A., Shirran, S. L., Botting, C. H. & Gates, M. A. Stathmin is enriched in the developing corticospinal tract. *Molecular and Cellular Neuroscience* **69**, 12–21 (2015).

78. Zhu, Y., Dou, M., Piehowski, P. D., Liang, Y., Wang, F., Chu, R. K., Chrisler, W. B., Smith, J. N., Schwarz, K. C., Shen, Y., Shukla, A. K., Moore, R. J., Smith, R. D., Qian, W. J. & Kelly, R. T. Spatially resolved proteome mapping of laser capture microdissected tissue with automated sample transfer to nanodroplets. *Molecular and Cellular Proteomics* **17**, 1864–1874 (2018).

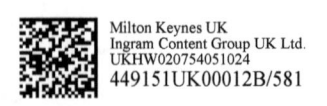

Milton Keynes UK
Ingram Content Group UK Ltd.
UKHW020754051024
449151UK00012B/581